TRUE
POWER
OF YOU

MARIOS SKARVELLIS

BALBOA.
PRESS
A DIVISION OF HAY HOUSE

Balboa Press books may be ordered through booksellers or by contacting:

Balboa Press
A Division of Hay House
1663 Liberty Drive
Bloomington, IN 47403
www.balboapress.com
1 (877) 407-4847

Print information available on the last page.

ISBN: 978-1-5043-7958-8 (sc)
ISBN: 978-1-5043-7957-1 (hc)
ISBN: 978-1-5043-7959-5 (e)

Library of Congress Control Number: 2017906266

Balboa Press rev. date: 05/10/2017

May the life essence be within you.

Acknowledge your achievements, be aware of your experiences, and give gratitude and praise to your failures and successes. These actions comprise the journey that unites mind, body, and spirit, which makes you complete with the true power of you, your creator, and the unity of the oneness.

My creative spirit consciousness, with the philosophy "energy flows where attention goes," allows the essence of the power of one to empower me and pursue with passion my inner awareness, insights, and knowledge of my essential body mechanics. It also lets me guide and support a global awareness to the collective world consciousness, maintaining the body's balanced alignment to enhance self-healing and encourage self-care, so as to achieve well-being and bring balance between mind, body, and spirit.

—Marios Skarvellis,
author, mind - body mentor,
life and success coach
www.truepowerofyou.com.au

energy flows where attention goes

CONTENTS

CHAPTER 1

SUCCESSFULLY OVERCOMING STRESS

My name is Marios Skarvellis. I am a mind - body mentor, a success coach, and a masseur. I have been studying human behavior and self-awareness techniques most of my life. I have found we collectively experience the same emotions – stress, depression, loneliness, and fears, but on different levels of awareness and attitude. I am deeply concerned about the mental health issues that affect us all. Mental health issues are discussed in all means of media and affect the young, the elderly, athletes, armchair observers, and intellects. No one escapes, and we all have a common enemy: our inner demons, which challenge us every moment of our lives.

In order to regularly have good thoughts, you need to make a conscious effort to create a new routine that supports a positive and optimistic outlook. Having negative thoughts and emotions comes easily; it's the default first response, because it is an immediate protection reflex, assuring one's safety, insecurities, and ego.

We are consumed by stress in all areas of our environment: work, home, and socially. Stress is the most talked about topic: what disappoints and upsets us, what people say and think about us, our insecurities and fears, the lack of respect and attention we get from others (whether it is friends or loved ones), and the big topic of finances.

The biggest "disease" we suffer from on this planet is through our own thoughts and emotions. Our negative self-talk and constant chatter on an everyday basis about the immediate thoughts and emotions that do not please us fuels this dis-ease. This constant chatter interferes with our normal mind-body communication and fuels our stress, anxiety, depression, fear, hate, anger, loneliness, and insecurity, which creates a feeling of separation from family, friends, and society, which also drives our addictions. Our minds communicate to our flesh-and-blood body machines through electromagnetic signals and biochemicals that are sent and received from every part of our bodies instantaneously, determining every action or movement we do.

Did you know that these negative thoughts and emotions increase the hormone Cortisol, which is produced by the central nervous system through biochemicals that are manifested and stored into our cellular and muscle memory. The result is tension, pain, and disease in our bodies. The effects of stress on the hormone cortisol also accelerate the aging process.

Stress lowers testosterone levels, and the majority of men's erectile problems are due to stress, low testosterone, and bad blood flow. A woman's estrogen and testosterone levels are also affected.

The mind and body need to have close communication in order to maintain well-being and true postural alignment. The human body was created to be in symmetry, to be in balance with itself, and to be in harmony with the energy and forces around it. If you improve your posture and alignment, you enhance movement, flexibility, and well-being. If I was to pinpoint one spot that affects postural alignment the most, it is the Achilles heel. There is a great deal of tension and strain placed on this point from regular foot movements. These tensions are transferred up your body tower and alter everything above, from your knee to you hip, spine, and neck. Every action has an equal and opposite reaction. Women wearing high-heeled shoes may look great, but they affect their Achilles heels by tightening them to a point where walking in flat shoes hurts. Women should be more aware and use heels only when required.

There is a positive or happy hormone, called endorphins. It's usually experienced during exercise, sex, laughing, and positive thoughts and emotions. These are some of the sources around which we can set new routines that will serve us.

Another biochemical, adrenalin, favours stressful activities associated with the energy and excitement of the fight-or-flight response. That is when you intentionally engage in a stressful or risky behavior for a self-inducing high. Becoming more aware and in control of our thoughts and emotions controls which biochemical we stimulate through our bodies every day, as well as how effectively our electromagnetic signals flow. When we begin awareness toward a mind-body communication that is in balance and harmony, we activate our physical instincts and sixth senses to their peak performance. This restores our bodies' natural energy field, or aura, to resonate at a true, individual, unique frequency, like an antenna.

Our bodies' true harmonic frequency (aura) connects to the universal flow of energy, which allows the power of attraction and intention into our lives. Where we place our attention is paramount to our well-being, longevity, happiness, and success. Remember that "Energy flows where attention goes." All our thoughts and emotions, whether happy or sad, good or bad, are connected and networked to every part of our bodies' cellular and muscle memory, sending and receiving information and commands that control and resonate throughout our bodies. Learning to be in control of our mind-body language and assuring they are positive and optimistic ones that assist and complement us every day, under any circumstances, is to our benefit and well-being; this increases our natural aura and sixth senses.

Your aura, your body's energy field, is collectively made up of seven major energy points, called chakras, and two energy lines that run parallel through your seven major joints. These chakras are located from the crown of your head through the centre of your body to the bottom of your pelvis, with the colours of the rainbow. The colours start from the bottom of your pelvis with red. These chakras are the true channels of communication to the soul, bringing balance to mind, body, and spirit. They need your constant awareness and nurturing in order to expand.

Did you know that 30–40 percent of your weight is from your skeletal frame, and that muscle weighs more than fat? So why are people so obsessed with weight when it comes to dieting? If you look lean and healthy, then you are lean and healthy no matter how much you weigh. The human body is made up of approximately 60 percent water, and the body composition varies according to gender and fitness levels, because fatty tissue contains less water than lean tissue. Your percentage of water also depends on your hydration level. You only begin to feel thirsty when you have already lost around 2–3 percent of your body's water. Mental performance and physical coordination start to become impaired before you become thirsty, and the body needs to be hydrated regularly. It is said that two liters a day is required for a healthy body to maintain well-being.

However, it is not common knowledge that forms of stress, anxiety, and more are subconsciously manifested into the body, having dehydrating effects on the body. Now add a common stress reliever or two, like cigarettes, coffee, soft drinks, alcohol, or drugs. They all have dehydrating effects on the body. If you are in the above category, the recommended two liters a day is not sufficient – you now require about three liters a day. The average person will drink about 1 liter a day or less, which is why a majority of people are dehydrated, causing tensing of muscle tissue and slower blood flow, that constricts the nervous system, which causes headaches, a pins and needles feeling, pain, lethargy and illness. If the body becomes dehydrated regularly, your cellular memory and muscle memory constricts, which affects your true alignment, balance, and symmetry.

Your subconscious auto protection system picks up on any tension in your body and tries to realign your body structure by shifting muscle mass to counterbalance any imbalance in your body. This affects your true alignment and the way you walk. A Japanese author and entrepreneur, Masaru Emoto, has written numerous books that claim the human consciousness has an effect on the molecular structure of water, of which we are 60 percent. Thoughts, emotions, and feelings are vibrations in our bodies, even affecting our heartbeat. Everything is based on energy frequencies that form vibrations all around us. These vibrations affect the water cells by altering the uniformed, balanced patterns they form. The higher the frequency, the more complex the patterns appear. Every frequency is an invisible wave of energy that emits a sound, however it's not one heard by normal hearing. A frequency has the ability to heal or harm you; you can virtually think yourself into illness. Emoto believes that water takes on the resonance of the energy which is directed at it. We are bombarded twenty-four seven every day by all types of frequencies and vibrations, and they affect our bodies' harmonic frequencies. Emoto also believes that polluted water can be restored through prayer, affirmations, and positive visualization: "Change the thought, change the feeling."

Our body machines are constantly at work, trying to stay at their peak performance. They are bombarded by viruses and diseases, and they carry out a preventative maintenance plan, especially when we are asleep. Every day the DNA in your body divides as many as two trillion times. Old cells die, and the body replaces them with duplicates. Even though these new duplicate cells are created, they are slightly less perfect than the original ones, which affects your aging. Keeping your DNA at its prime, peak performance at all times allows you to be healthier, happier, more vibrant, and more confident every day.

Have you ever noticed how people walk? I would like you to take a moment to become aware of your movements, by observing how you and other people move. You will notice how one or both legs turn outward like a penguin. I encourage you to become more aware and focus on the placement of your feet. Persist in straightening your feet so your foundations can be stable again. Your mind processes all new information to address anything out of balance, and it can set new default alignments that do not always serve you and put you further out of balance. Your mind uses the information it receives to create new results and outcomes. By looking down as you are walking and becoming aware of how you place your feet down – heel to toe, with pressure more on the inner heel and the big toe – you give your brain new realignment settings that serve your well-being and balance.

This may be uncomfortable at first, but pain is something we live with every day. Whether we are totally aware of it or not, it still lies within our bodies and only becomes aware to us when someone touches us, or we put our bodies through a strenuous action. As they say, no pain, no gain.

Face your pain and release it. Use your attention and awareness, to improve your personal development and self-care. Look within the darkness of your subconscious mind where energy flows, where attention goes. There are many habits, routines, and beliefs that our collective world conscious has handed down from ancestor to ancestor, and today they do not serve us and have weakened our mind, body, and spirit symmetry. One of them was a strict upbringing of using your right hand, and punishing and ridiculing those who used their left hand. That has left our population mainly using the right hand instinctively, rather than encouraging an ambidextrous point of view. People who are ambidextrous are uncommon, only one in one hundred.

Our creator, God, fashioned the blueprint of a male and female earthling, using a Homo sapiens design you know – the skeletal frame we see at Halloween and doctors' offices. The design was equal and in balance left and right, and it supported an inner feature for balance and symmetry. Over thousands of years, we have inadvertently and subconsciously altered our DNA, our cellular and muscle memory, to one that is not in balance with itself or the outer forces of energy.

Our minds use the subconscious DNA files handed down from our parents and ancestors that define our characteristics and parameters as a human being. Our minds also rely on the information of our natural five senses for decision making and actions. We may not be at fault for where we are today as earthlings, but we are definitely responsible for our future and the next generation. It is up to each and every one of us, to improve and reeducate our self-care and personal development, in order to restore the true power of humankind. We are all intuitive beings; it's only our physicality that gets in the way. We have to remember that we are living spiritual beings in physical bodies, and we have roles to play other than our egos and attitudes controlling our lives. We need to stand up and be accountable for our actions and our future.

May the essence be within you.

CHAPTER 2

YOUR LIFE VEHICLE

The human body is a intricately complex living machine, a flesh-and-blood life vehicle that is your transporter. It is like a robot with a far more intricate design, and it is very loyal and obedient without judgment. When it's guided, nurtured, and loved, it works to its peak performance, drawing on all its resources and processing skills for your disposal. It has a logical and analytical processing system based on probabilities; that's how regularly and often you think and do things, and your repetitious routines become habits.

It uses default subconscious files from your ancestors' DNA to define your appearance, habits, routines, beliefs, and attitudes. Your body machine's seven major joints allow its flexibility, and your five physical senses provide data so you can move through all environments and situations. Your life vehicle takes you – the self-consciousness ego with your life essence's inner spirit consciousness, which is the power source to your life vehicle – wherever you want to go, under any circumstance and in any environment.

Each of the seven major joints is supported by muscle fibers that have a muscle memory, supporting every angle of the joint. Joints can move in a circular motion clockwise and anticlockwise, however, we mainly use an up-and-down movement in our everyday sedentary movements.

Many fibers combine to create a muscle. Each muscle has a muscle memory, and every thought and emotion you have affects your muscle memory. If you feel happy, positive, optimistic, and loved, then your body feels better and works better for you. If your thoughts and emotions are negative, unhappy, disappointing, angry, and jealous, then there will be tension and pain in your muscle memory and body. Your thoughts and emotions will automatically affect the muscle memory around your seven joints, and any slight changes on your joints will affect your postural alignment. Our brain-mind-body communication processes information from every spot in our bodies, sending and receiving information instantaneously. This mind-body communication is a part of our automatic blueprint and programming by our creator as part of the design for a human.

Learning to work with our automatic mind-body communication allows us to improve our physiology and well-being. Every human needs to learn how to master his or her mind-body communication skills.

It is our responsibility to improve ourselves as individuals, and it begins with self-awareness, self-development, self-control, and self-care. These factors lead to your self-healing.

Our minds depend on new information and knowledge to process for our creativity and self-development, and they rely on our five natural physical senses: hearing, sight, touch, smell, and taste. That way we can move through our various environments every day, whether it be at work, with family, with friends, or in unknown environments.

Our hearing through our eardrums detects vibrations, sounds, and frequencies. Our sight through our eyes detects colour and light to interpret our environment by focusing and detecting images. Our touch through our skin detects pain, pressure, and temperatures. Our smell through our noses detects scents and odors. Our taste through our tongues detects sweet, salty, sour, and bitter, which are based off chemical reactions. Our brains also gather information from our subconscious ancestral DNA files and our self-conscious ego files. That includes files that do not always serve us, like fears, phobias, anxiety, depression, and diseases. We're processing all of them twenty-four seven with every decision we make. The brain's processing system is far superior to any computers on this planet. Whatever information we allow our brains to regularly process is what outcome we will create. One of God's given assets is the power of free will, and it's a power that needs to be mastered and controlled.

Our constant self-chatter can be our best friend or our worst enemy. This self-chatter has regularly been conditioned to focus on things that have or will make us unhappy, disappoint us, or upset us. Usually it's about money, relationships, and career, leaving our immediate thoughts and emotions focused on negative ones. The more negative thoughts and emotions our minds have to process, the deeper they lead us to stress, anxiety, depression, suicide, and many more mental health issues.

We need to become aware of our self-chatter and choose wisely regarding what we think about every day. Collectively, every day builds to every week and then every month, forming negative attitudes that attract negative actions toward us, affecting us with many mood swings. As we know, life has its ups and downs, however we are responsible for them. Our creator gave us the power of free will, and whatever we think we can create and we can alter.

It is imperative to become aware with full intention to what you are truly thinking and what you truly want. Do your habits serve and assist you daily? For every thought, there is an emotion attached to it, and to every emotion, there is a thought attached to it. Choose your thoughts and control your emotions wisely. Design your life around positive intensions.

We have always heard about good and bad, right and wrong, positive and negative outcomes, however we have not understood how much influence we have over them. "Energy flows where attention goes." Where we place our attention and focus determines our outcomes. Thinking of things that we don't want in our life regularly attracts those things to us; this is negative thinking.

Have gratitude and appreciate what you have. Focus on what you want and believe that you will get it. Have faith in God's design and stay optimistic with all your thoughts and emotions, and you will attract them to you. You are God's unique design, a blueprint design manual of a human. Within this blueprint default manual is knowledge, and within this knowledge is power, as well as unknown secrets you can tap into for your self-healing and well-being.

In order to access all we desire, we need to improve our mind-body communication and postural alignment. This will get us close up and personal with our true power source, our sixth senses. By using our essential body mechanics and the seven major joints as reference points, we improve our mind-body awareness. With regular focus and repetitive attention, it presents us with our own preventative maintenance program, which I call Destressercise.

Destressercise is a preventative maintenance program that runs automatically through our existing, default mind-body processing system. By becoming more aware of our mind-body communication, it allows us to access this system to self-educate and

17

fine-tune our mind-body communication skills. Our bodies' posture has been modified from the original creation. The life vehicle we call a human body was designed by the creator to be in balance and symmetry with itself. Our transporter was designed for us to gain information through experiences, knowledge, and awareness of our surroundings, and we can store this information in our subconscious memory banks for future use. The gathering of knowledge and storing this information as memory in our DNA spirit energy files is a part of the legacy to fulfill our ancestral destiny. The combination of present and past ancestral memory files and our original blueprint creator's default memory files, allows our ever-expanding life essence spirit to continue its growth and evolution into the life essence virtual reality that God designed. Our human bodies' blueprint design was programmed to protect us and never harm itself. It listens to all our commands and is available to us at all times. Only from the self-consciousness can the ego harm us and our life vehicles. We have to respect and appreciate our life vehicles for them to be at there peak performance and to give us longevity, youthfulness, happiness, and well-being.

Stress is the biggest disease or (dis-ease) on the planet, and it affects all humans. We have allowed stress and negative talk to enter our self-chatter and fester into our mental demons, causing mental health issues that consume our planet and form physical illnesses like heart attacks, strokes, cancer, and many other issues.

In order to successfully overcome stress, we need to change our emotional attitude toward stress. We need to control our negative emotions and thoughts to ensure optimistic and positive outcomes. We need to use hindsight as an example of our past, how our emotional state has misled and misguided us to make incorrect decisions, and how there were always other options to handle situations that arise.

To fulfill your life's destiny, remember this line: "Energy flows where attention goes." You need to get close up and personal with your body machine and muscle memory. Getting close contact to your muscle memory is the first step to taking back full control of your life vehicle. Imagine that the body you look at in the mirror is your machine. Look it in the eyes and say hello with respect, confidence, trust, and love. Then say, "I would like to know you. Will you please help me? I am trying to access my operations manual so I can know all your features and can access my DNA files. If necessary, I would like to change them."

The life vehicle's brain processes a direct command from you, the self-consciousness, the ego, to access your subconscious files. Your brain has never heard you make this request before, so it needs regular and repetitive assurance this is really what you want. If you do not request access again, your life vehicle will not respond because it has a default setting that is programmed to do what its regular habits, routines, and beliefs are. You need to control the inner chatter and the external chatter to have full control. The outer chatter is what you say to others; you need to walk the talk, say and do what your real intentions are. Your outer chatter can also be used while on your own in front of a mirror, where you can communicate directly eye to eye with yourself in order to obtain a great deal of information about your life vehicle's posture, flexibility, youthfulness, confidence, habits, and routines. You need to check on the condition of your life vehicle to get your optimal and best performance at all times. You need to tune it in. You are your worst enemy and best friend; treat yourself the way you want others to treat you, respect yourself, and help yourself like a friend, lover, or family member. Go out of your way to please your life vehicle, and even get intimate and passionate with it. It has been given to you by God for this life experience; get to know it and take a ride into your future. Think of what you truly want in life. Set a goal toward it and keep heading that way. You as the ego need to believe that every outcome ahead of you is not a failure, setback, or mistake, but a step toward what you want. Assess where you are at anytime in your life: "What is the next best thing toward gaining my goal?"

To attain your goal, it all works through the power of intention, good or bad. They say that karma's a bitch, and it's true. If you go forth with good intentions to your goal, you will find the least resistant way there. Everything is a test on achieving your enlightenment and getting closer to your source, God, our creator. There is a bit of reality in everything you know and have seen, because our collective world virtual reality consciousness has become aware of it, sharing it with others, that creates a new belief, philosophy, or fantasy on this planet.

Our planet is the Garden of Eden that is mentioned by scribes in the Bible. Heaven, purgatory, and hell are all here; it simply depends on which one you feed the most with your thoughts and emotions.

Evil, black magic, Satan – all exist on this planet. They are a part of our collective world virtual reality consciousness, and each of us has the power of free will, so we have given the dark energy life.

Satan is the leader of all our inner demons, and as we feed our inner demons, we destroy ourselves and our very existence. You have heard of the all-seeing eye? That is God, who is within us and all around us – not the big brother system that spies on us all. However, for thousands of years, there has been another eye; in Greek it's called the *mati*, or *matiasma*, the evil eye. Evil people who focus words, evil thoughts, and emotions into incantations toward you can place a curse or spell on you. The power of free will, when used incorrectly, is very evil. You can unintentionally wish bad things to befall others, and gossip of envy or jealous admiration from the support of others can bring harm upon people. Be wise, humane, and respectful of your powers. God has not forsaken us. We have chosen to walk the talk with evil intentions, attracting evil outcomes.

Our creator created the Garden of Eden with all its unique designs for us to explore, enjoy, nurture, and guide our evolution into the future, in order to pass on to the next generation a preserved garden that sustains life for our existence with all we need to live within it. God only asks for us to stay close and have faith in the creator's designs.

We have misunderstood the story of Adam and Eve, the blueprint to all male and female earthlings. They were supposedly enticed by the snake to take the apple from the tree of knowledge so they could become gods themselves. God had already made them creators of their own, blessing them with the power of free will. The snake was representing wisdom, faith, and healing, warning Adam and Eve that feeding on the apple from the tree of knowledge required awareness and responsibility for its power, and that knowledge alone, with the power of free will, would harm and destroy them. This was a warning that the power of knowledge and the power of free will bestowed upon them by God, with their own logical and analytical ego, that it would distract them from there natural instincts and pull them away from their sixth senses and their creator.

This is where we have evolved today. We have distanced ourselves from our creator with many manmade doctrines called religion. God has always been there within us. He has not forsaken us, because with the power of free will, we can reconnect the bond. It's time, and we must choose the correct path to restore the balance of good and bad energy on our planet and the true power of one. You make a difference. It starts with believing and having faith, because collectively we are the world consciousness. If we all focus on the good, love, happiness, respect, and honour, it strengthens our very existence.

CHAPTER 3

OUR CREATOR

Our creator has spent infinity evolving from the energy of the dark matter, which is dark space, to the essence of life and the Holy Spirit energy. The creator fashioned the life essence virtual reality designs in the book of creations, the book of life. Like a child with crayons and a blank page, the squiggles and lines took formation, and the cosmos was shaped and formed to produce movement, vibration, frequencies, and magnetic fields, which formed a unique resonance to allow his designs to hold these default settings. The pages are the dark space we see in the sky at night. The lights are our creator's unique designs, the planets and galaxies that form the cosmos.

Our creator formed a resonance, a life essence frequency that would network all life creations as one essence of life. Everything in the cosmos works to precision and clockwork, not missing a beat in an infinite and timeless universe. The planets have unique environments, sizes, orbits, speeds, chemical balances, and rotations within a galaxy, and each galaxy is networked to another, forming the cosmos like spider webs grouped together. Nothing is by accident; it is a divine design made up of a network of magnetic fields and frequencies that resonate through the cosmos and that allow all of God's designs to be defined and evolved, so that every planet can hold its default settings and remains in its own set orbit.

Our ancestors believed that the earth was the centre of our galaxy, and they were right. It's not in the centre like a dartboard, but everything in our galaxy. Every planet, moon, and star was formed and set in motion with its own individual defaults, to serve and provide for our creator's living planet, Earth.

Any objects that are broken from these default settings set by God and are in a out-of-control orbit (meteor, comet, etc.) is due to some imbalance of the resonating frequencies in the cosmos. Every action has an equal and opposite reaction, and it reacts and reflects upon everything in the cosmos. Why are we so afraid of the unknown? Why does everything have to be proven to be accepted? There are many things we do not have all the answers to, and still we accept them: our instincts, our gut feeling, our intuitiveness, our self-healing powers, love, our very existence, the endless cosmos, and other life forms. Do you really think a designer like our creator would make us and every other design on this planet with so much colour and variety without repeating it somewhere in the cosmos?

The birth of a child takes eight to nine months to produce a living being, a future creator with sixth senses and the power of free will. This is a miracle. Everything we know and everything we do is a part of God's designs, which are available to us to find and which we become aware of and evolve into. Every great invention, theory, and philosophy is already in our subconscious life essence spirit files, awaiting to be discovered; we simply need faith and belief in our creator's designs.

Any creative design needs passion, determination, enthusiasm, faith, belief and the right attitude to be discovered. Every day, something is discovered,

27

innovated, and modified to provide us with a new idea or philosophy for a easier and simpler lifestyle. Wow, we really do underestimate our creator! We are descendants of the pure oneness, where there is no resistance, forever expanding and evolving timelessly. The creator has big plans for the expansion of the life essence, so with the spirit of the essence of life, he designed his life beings, his earthlings, to also be creators and assist in the evolution and expansion of life in the cosmos. We are children in the universe; our creator asks only for you to have faith and believe in the designs fashioned and placed in the book of creations.

We have not mentally, physically, or spiritually evolved into an enlightenment of spirituality that has no limitations. God did not encourage or ask for manmade religions, politics, nationalities, wars, famine, and diseases to consume his living planet and living beings. Our ancestors created all of these, and it is up to us as individuals to find our true paths back to our creator and the true power of ourselves, which lies deep within the souls of our life vehicles. Start your journey and may the essence be within you.

As we have been told, man was made in the image of the creator, God. However, our creator is not of the physical image. We were created from the same essence of life from which he evolved, an essence of life that is pure matter, pure energy, pure spirit. It is a spirit that has been evolving for a long time, where time as we know it doesn't even exist. We need to have faith in God and his earthling design. Within his life vehicle's soul, he bestowed his spirit, his essence of life, so he would be connected to us and all his life beings.

Our creator commenced by forming an environment, a living planet of living beings of all levels of existence, to coexist in harmony and balance in his Garden of Eden. We know it as the living planet, Earth, a blueprint to all life in the cosmos. Each earthling is unique in its own way, the same but different. We were conditioned to fit into our creator's Garden of Eden because all life beings are part of the life essence spirit energy. We are one with everything, every unique design resonating its own frequency. At the first meeting of his earthlings and life beings with Mother Nature, Father Sky, and creation, our divine purpose was to fuse into our environment with love, respect, dignity, leadership, and direction to nurture and connect all life. We should listen and grow, gather data to analyze, review and store all data memory, and design and create the evolution of life. We should learn the feelings of love, a united, collective network that bonds us mentally, physically, and spiritually to God. We are now his creators, assisting in nurturing, guiding, protecting, and admiring all of the other life beings down to their very cells, in order to appreciate Mother Nature's insects, animals, and other earthlings. We are all one.

Our creator loves variety. There are six hundred species of animals on this planet, and each species has thousands of flying creatures, land creatures, and ocean creatures of all shapes and sizes and colours. Mother Nature has a wide variety of forests and jungles and deserts. The list goes on and on. Off the planet, there are endless galaxies with unknown creatures. All the great designs God fashioned are reproduced, modified, and reused in the book of creations.

We marvel at our software writers on this planet for the great programs they produce: office packages, games, programs that simplify our lives. Virtual reality that makes us feel totally engrossed in the images. We feel a part of them, and they can deceive our physical senses.

However, we underestimate our creator, who designed the ultimate virtual reality 3-D life experience that we live in. It is time we appreciate and respect what we have been given, what our creator has bestowed upon us, and who we really are. It's a power that we only use a minute percentage of, and our destiny is not to be mere mortals but to be immortals. We are earthlings, and we have to believe it's true and possible before we can achieve it.

Now is our time to begin a new era for humanity. We are not just humans; we have to restore ourselves on the planet, in the galaxy, and in the cosmos as earthlings. It's our responsibility as individuals to do our bit and to make the planet, our place to live, as one of peace. One for all, and all for one – this is our destiny. The human being, our blueprint, is a Homo sapiens design that all humans share. This common design makes us all earthlings. No matter what we look like externally or believe in, our DNA, our building blocks, are all cells that evolved from an essence of life. Every cell, no matter how minute, has a role to play in the big picture. Each cell has a memory that is connected by resonating frequencies, which network all life essences together. Everything affects everything, and no matter how minor it is, the connection is there. We are a major factor of the in balance on our planet. We radiate an energy field around us, an aura. Our aura is strong when our inner spirit and outer spirit are connected. Just like our planet has its aura, the ozone layer, but the planet is only as strong as the collective energy made up of all the living beings within it.

We are responsible for getting everything back on track and reconnecting with our creator. God has not forsaken us, and he is the soul within us, our true power source. He has always been there for us; we simply choose not to see or understand how it all works. We prefer to blame God for everything rather than take responsibility for our actions, ignoring the power of free will and the effects it has on everything.

The power of free will and our sixth senses are a gift from God. The apple from the tree of knowledge represents the physical, analytical, and logical powers of our mind. The Lucifer effect, the snake, represents spiritual healing and our sixth senses who warned Adam and Eve that with knowledge there is power, and it needs to be used wisely.

Our creator warned us not to drift too far away from his spirit, or else our inner demons would control us. Our creator left us a manual, and it lies within us. We need to connect with our inner Holy Spirit energy, and in order to do that, we need to recognize and become aware of our seven major energy chakra points, which run through our body and expand our aura, our antenna, to resonate the correct magnetic frequency so that the power of intention and attraction work correctly for us.

Everything that our creator has created and fashioned in the book of creations is based on the eternal circle. Wherever you start on a circle, it ends and restarts again endlessly. Every cell, every planet, every galaxy – everything is networked by the movement of circles, rotating, orbiting in our creator's Holy Spirit energy network. We are all bound to each other. There is no missing link in man's evolution. Like any great designer, a new design can be improvised and improved with leaps and bounds: Homo erectus, the animals, and Mother Nature formed the prehistoric design. God was not satisfied with that, and so the evolution of all God's creations is part of a divine design. He erased it, but like all his designs, it is not destroyed but placed in another dimension, or page of the book of creations. Our continents did not break away by accident; it was by divine force. Our creator divided the continents. He also created the Homo sapiens design, his blueprint for all his future earthlings.

God loves a variety of designs, and so fashioned many different earthlings with different colours, sizes, languages, cultures, habits, routines, and characteristics to fit in many different environments. Our creator planned that one day, our spiritual bond and physical curiosity would draw us to each other, and we'd become aware of each other and offer each other new ideas, philosophies, beliefs, respect, and love. We would work together to evolve as a greater earthling, an immortal. The power of free will was and is our greatest challenge, and it's an overwhelming desire and a lust for power. We became selfish, greedy, and envious. With knowledge there is power in our physical world. Our mental self-chatter consumed us, allowing the power of our mental demons to take us further away from our sixth senses and our connection with God.

Our creator has always had faith in us to find our way back, because he is within us and all around us. Let's step out of our brain and let our natural instincts guide us back to the creator's blueprint that fashioned life vehicles with a self-consciousness and his spiritual image within. We're meant to be part of the Garden of Eden, the life planet, and to be nurturers and gardeners in order to protect, guide, and evolve the life essence. We are still young in the evolution of the universe, however a time for our change and enlightenment is close to us. It is a time where we can, as the power of one, receive the energy at a peak time in our solar system. The year is 2018. We need our energy antennas to be in tune. We must begin the preparations and awareness to restore our place on our planet and in the cosmos.

May the essence be within you.

CHAPTER 4

THE SEVEN MAJOR CHAKRAS

Your seven major chakras are energy points that strategically lie in the soul of your life vehicle. If they are all in balance, they form an energy field around your life vehicle, which is your aura, strengthening your sixth senses and resonating a frequency that allows the power of free will, the power of intention, and the power of attraction to complete your destiny.

The chakras run from the bottom of your life vehicle, grounding you spiritually with the essence of life to Mother Earth and up through your body to the top of your head and out, to Father Sky, before going back to Mother Nature, completing the circle of life.

Each chakra is made up of energy circles in the colours of the rainbow. When our inner and outer spirit energies are aligned and in frequency, our seven energy chakras are strong, giving us a strong aura that resonates the required frequency for the true power of us to be revealed. I remember in science that white light refracting through a clear pyramid giving us the colours of the rainbow, just like light refracts through rain drops in the sky to create a real rainbow. I still use a name that my teacher gave us to remember the sequence of the rainbow colours: it was ROY. G. BIV.

Starting from the bottom, your first chakra is the letter R, representing the colour red. Your base chakra is located around the groin area, the vital organs for birth and life, grounding and connecting you to Mother Nature and all living beings. As you move up to the second chakra point, between your groin and naval button is your essential chakra. The letter O represents orange, which connects you to your intimacy with life and all beings.

The third chakra is located at your naval button; the letter Y represents the colour yellow, your main chakra. The naval chakra is where you were connected to your mother by an umbilical cord, and where all the ancestral DNA memory and Holy Spirit energy was passed on to you. You were activated to evolve as the person you have now become. The fourth is the heart chakra and is located at the same level as your heart, but in the centre of your chest. The letter G represents the colour green, which connects you with your emotions, good or bad. The fifth is your throat chakra, located at your throat. The letter B represents the colour blue and connects you through communication and knowledge to everything around you.

The sixth is your third eye chakra. The letter I represents the colour indigo, and it is located between your eyes and directly above your nose. This is your all-seeing eye, connecting you with your inner and outer spirit energies. The seventh is your crown chakra. The letter V represents the colour violet. It is located at the top of your head and connects you to your outer spirit energy.

Awareness of each of these energy chakras, and regular attention and focus to their locations and colours, strengthens them. When sitting in a quiet place with your eyes shut, focus on each one individually. Then from the ground chakra, you draw Mother Nature within your very being, up through all your chakras and out through your crown, up to Father Sky and then back down to your base chakra again, on the left and right side of your body at the same time. The process forms a magnetic field of energy that creates the circles of life, where the beginning and the end are at the same place – the eternal circle of life. When all seven chakras are in balance and aligned, your aura is at its peak performance and resonates the true frequency that makes you more than a mere mortal; it connects you to your sixth sense. This is not difficult for you to do, but you have to become aware of the seven points. Focus on them and practice daily. Remember that energy flows where attention goes.

When your life vehicle, the human body, dies, your inner Holy Spirit energy networks all your ancestral DNA memory to the collective Holy Spirit energy, allowing all your gathered life knowledge and experiences to continue and evolve, as our creator has set in motion from generation to generation. If we do not regularly cleanse ourselves mentally, physically, or spiritually, we become too stagnant, lost, and lonely within ourselves. The majority of our lives is disconnected from Mother Nature, our spiritual bond to this planet and our creator. We are becoming more engrossed with old doctrines and technology, focusing too much on everything around us in our everyday lives. We have forgotten how to connect with God, our creator, from within. We need to become more aware of the mind, body, and spirit balance. There has to be a balance between all in order for us to be at our peak performance. We need to spiritually balance our chakras, and we need a good communication mentally and physically. We should spend more time in nature, because we have disconnected ourselves from all of God's designs.

May the essence be within you.

CHAPTER 5

THE TRUE POWER OF YOU

The true power of you is the ultimate virtual reality mind game, where you have the power of free will and the philosophy that "Energy flows where attention goes." By focusing and becoming aware of your sixth chakra, which is the colour indigo and is your third eye, you begin your journey by entering the darkness of the unknown. It's a journey that gets you close up and personal with the true power of you.

Imagine you are a spiritual warrior, like a Jedi Knight. You have a yellow light saber as your faith, your mission, to enter a space, where the energy of the dark forces and your mental demons dwell. It's a journey that takes you on an adventure of a lifetime, that defies reality as you find the ultimate prize that has eluded man for thousands of years. You can finally find your true power source, access the tree of knowledge, drink from the fountain of youth, and restore your sixth senses. It's a journey only you can take, alone, and with knowledge there is power.

Find the secrets, tools, and weapons that allow you to become aware of the true power of you and your sixth senses. The truth may be out there, but it's quicker if you go deep within the soul of your flesh-and-blood body machine in order to find all you desire, so you can conquer your demons. Like any journey, there are always obstacles and difficulties to overcome, as well as some pain to tolerate and endure. Are you prepared to begin your ultimate challenge and face your inner demons and fears in order to restore your strength and faith in the true power of you?

Enter your third eye and go into the darkness. Get yourself close up and personal with the Jedi warrior and the true potential of your power. Feel your mind, body, and spirit unite as one. Gather your strength and power. Draw your light saber, raise your weapon, and face your demons. Have faith in the essence of life and God, and find the life essence spirit energy force that lies within you. Never give in, never give up, and absolutely never surrender to your inner demons. May the essence be within you!

I am a reflection of my source, which is magnificent in all ways. So why has all of our history been based on individuals struggling for power and control over the masses? These people striving for power and control, preventing a true unity between us all as a world consciousness, use the evil eye to stop us from accessing our sixth senses and stagnate the true power of humankind. They have used wars, diseases, media outlets, subliminal messages on TV, and songs to condition human beings into insecurities, fears, anxieties, stresses, beliefs, routines, and habits that disconnect them from Mother Nature and do not serve them mentally, physically, or spiritually as individuals or as a world consciousness.

The unity of the human race is our birthright. It is in our DNA makeup, and it is an energy that sustains the essence of life and the source to our divine power: the power of one, which is the power of you and the power of all living beings, networked to evolve into the true destiny in the life essence. From the blueprint and DNA of our existence and all living beings comes a birthright that once had us all side by side, working for a common cause. It is an energy that all living beings possess, like beacons, like stars radiating unique energy fields. We have our own auras, our natural networks of communication between each essence of life.

It's a natural gift bestowed upon all life by the creator. Our sixth senses are our intuitive, psychic, creative, maternal instincts, and paternal instincts. They are far more than our five physically conscious senses.

Our five physically conscious senses are constantly collecting data, parameters, and information that assist our physical bodies to function in every environment. Our hearing, sight, smell, touch, and taste are part of an auto consciousness programming system that receives, analyses, and stores all records into our intricate, vast subconscious filing system, which runs the human body or life vehicle without self-conscious (ego) participation or awareness. These records help form our physiology (posture) routines, habits, and beliefs without our awareness.

For centuries, we have been conditioned to suppress our natural sixth senses, our true godly powers. In ancient times, many men and woman healers and leaders followed the path of nature and were in tune with its forces. They had the knowledge of herbs and medicines and gave wise counsel. They were held in high esteem and knew that what they took from Mother Nature they would returned in some way to maintain the balance and equilibrium of the forces. Today we have put an imbalance in Mother Nature, causing many natural catastrophes.

In the Bible and in many other doctrines, the creator fashioned man and woman from his own image. This was not a physical image, but the essence of life that he evolved from. It's the same spirit of the essence of life that is within you and all living beings; it's the same essence of life that connects all life essences as one with the creator. The bond can never be broken. Even when the physical human body that houses and protects your inner spirit dies, your inner spirit is restored to it true source, the creator, the essence of life that will always continue evolving into the energy of the dark matter (space), which is the base for all life. By reactivating our natural godly senses, we help restore our true resonances and frequencies collectively into the universe. That resonance and frequency is currently weak and out of harmony and balance with the universe and our creator.

The human body, our life vehicles, our transporters, had a malfunction thousands of years ago. Our auto conscious sped up the intake of negative data, information, and knowledge at an alarming rate, causing an overload. It did not leave adequate intervals for our sixth senses to assist and guide us as we were created to function, suppressing our natural, instinctive abilities to a small fraction of their capability.

As our self-conscious, our ego, our character traits also evolved through our ancestors' DNA cellular memories of physiology, beliefs, habits, routines, thoughts, emotions, and characteristics, our self-talk constant chatter on issues, doubts, and fears consumed our thoughts and emotions, assisting in the suppression of our natural senses and instincts.

Our self-conscious, our egos, are not totally in control of our lives. Our subconscious runs on the files preprogrammed and stored from our mothers and fathers, from ancestral DNA information that is deciphered and determines our actions based on what percentage of information is in each file.

They cover each and every subject of life and will be logically prioritized, analyzed, and gathered by the auto consciousness to determine our responses to every thought and emotion we experience.

The human being is made up of a number of consciousnesses and data that allows the human part to function as an individual, a family member, a friend, a worker, and a member of our life planet. However, the *being* part is the spirit of the essence of life that is housed within the human body. Like a computer, the subconscious is a database and filing system that stores every bit of information from every point of the body's organs and nervous system, with every experience you've had every day of your life, as well as all information passed down from your ancestors' DNA cellular memory. There are intricate and in-depth files on everything, and no memory is erased, but stored in files to which you may not have access. The auto conscious is the ongoing processor that works twenty-four seven and allows all commands to proceed as the files are stored.

For example, we have all either driven or walked a regular journey we are familiar with, and we can find ourselves daydreaming about a favourite pastime.

However the auto conscious will complete the journey that is stored in our subconscious without our conscious participation. Then when we become aware we are at the end of the journey, and we do not remember the common things we see on that journey normally. We find it hard to believe how we got there. This happens in every action we do – eating, walking, and taking are not self-conscious commands; they are auto conscious commands that we regularly do in our sedentary movements, in the same manner, style, or tone.

Your self-conscious constantly challenges your logical thoughts with your emotional thoughts, allowing you to be impulsive and not always do the logical, rational choice. Your self-conscious constantly puts doubts in your mind: should you or shouldn't you, yes or no, right or wrong, love or hate. There is your self-awareness that we do not use regularly, because your self-conscious and auto conscious take priority over your subconscious files, so you are not always aware of your true physical and mental parameters.

Our mind-body communication is not in line with the true blueprint design that the creator set. We need to get into the control panel and set some

new parameters for our subconscious files to use as a new set point. For example, stand at attention like you are in the army as a soldier, and become aware of where specifically you feel tension, pain, and out of balance, so that new information and parameters can be processed rather than the ones that do not always serve you from your self-conscious and past ancestors' files.

Self-conscious and past ancestor memory filing works off probabilities of regularities and commonalities that get filed together, Your mum and dad may have medical issues that are hereditary, and you may or may not have the same issues. It depends on how the memories of all your ancestors correlated your DNA sequences when you were born. No two humans can ever be the same exactly, even twins, however all the DNA memory is still inside your memory banks from every ancestor and beyond. We may not be the direct cause to our human dilemma with each other, Mother Nature, Father Sky, all other living beings, and our connection to the endless universe. However, we are responsible for altering and undoing the changes required to receive the correct frequency that will restore us to our true destiny and get us close up and personal with our inner creator. Let the true power of you be a legacy to all mankind, all living beings, this is your journey into the life essence.

We are complex human beings that have not reached even a fraction of our potential. It is time we took back control of our life vehicle its self-care in order to allow our natural self-healing, self-immune, self-protect, and self-alignment systems to work at their peak performance, bringing balance to our minds, bodies, and spirits so that they can work in harmony, as they were fashioned to.

As balance is restored to human beings, our antennas and our frequencies resonate out, increasing our energy fields. With our true auras restored, we are again connected to the energy of the creator, bringing harmony to all living beings and our life planet's aura, the ozone layer. We as human beings do make a difference, and we are the key to restoring the essence of life, as we were intended to do. The journey begins with the power of us taking back control of our life vehicles' parameters and processing system. Sounds daunting? Not at all. The true power of you is the fountain of youth that restores our longevity, well-being, self-healing, self-protect, self-immunity, and intuitive powers that lie within us. Our lives have been constantly focused on what is happening around us and how we can fit in and belong. We have forgotten to look after our natural, God-given creative powers.

We are more than we seem. Our thoughts and emotions determine our futures. All through history, great people have added a part of themselves that has shifted and moved the collective environment or world consciousness, achieving feats of strength, endurance, intuitiveness, inventions, and discoveries that have altered our perspective of our achievements as human beings. Who remembers Jules Verne and *Twenty Thousand Leagues under the Sea*? It was a fiction book, like many written over history, in a time where only sailboats were our means of transport over the ocean. His imagination created a submarine with all kinds of technology and gear for man to walk underwater, and it had not been invented yet. God has provided us with an unlimited creative consciousness. Today, while reading that book, our awareness is that it's normal; there are submarines in many navies, and the technology is commonplace. The great Leonardo da Vinci was an inventor who designed planes and helicopters, and in the medical world he was the main person to start intricate recording of the human body, dissecting dead bodies at a time where it was heresy. He was an artist, sculptor, architect, mathematician, philosopher, and astrologist. He allowed his creativity to run wild through his connection with his sixth senses.

Let's look to more recent times. George Lucas and the Star Wars movies involve traveling through space, with creatures from other planets interacting with human beings. All are connected to the Force, and Jedi Knights can use the Force to perform supernatural fetes. The light saber is activated by the Jedi's oneness with the Force, the energy of the life essence, allowing them to perform at their peak performance as peacekeepers. May the Force be with you – or as I say, may the essence be within you.

Each one of us has the creative power of one, the power of you. At peak performance, we can contribute to the expansion, development, and reactivation of the evolution of the life essence. The creator formed a creative God consciousness so that all he created in the book of creations would be available to all of us to manifest as part of the evolution of the life essence virtual reality.

Like a child, God began a journey for the evolution of the essence of life to begin. He let the energy of his creative thoughts and emotions form a memory, a life essence memory that is required to sustain any cell of life.

CHAPTER 6

YOUR SIXTH SENSES

We are earthlings, and the human side is our life vehicle. It has five physical senses. The *being* side is our Holy Spirit energy, which is made up of two spiritual senses. The sixth sense is your instincts, intuition, psychic ability, creativity, and self-healing powers. The sixth sense is not of the physical being but is housed within the soul of the physical being. The life vehicle has become the soul that has cut the natural, harmonic communication between the inner spirit and our outer life essence spirit energy due to our logical and analytical thinking and our emotional ego. We have misused the power of free will that our creator bestowed upon us, allowing inner demons and emotions to control us, cutting our harmonic frequency to our creator. We have been conditioned in our life vehicles by the DNA memory handed down from ancestor to ancestor, from generation to generation, wanting to control everything through our logical and analytical self-consciousness, needing to prove everything before we can believe it. Our creative fantasy world has been affected, and our imagination still runs wildly through movies and books, but we are restricted by our lack of connection and understanding of our sixth senses – ones that connect us directly with our creator.

Through our constant thirst for power, control, and manipulation over other human beings, animals, and Mother Nature, our enlightenment has diminished, and we have jammed the natural harmonics that were resonating. Therefore we need to realign our physical antennas to resonate at the right frequency in order to be in balance with our life vehicles and the life essences within us, as well as the essence of life trying to connect with us.

Our seventh spiritual sense is when we leave our physical bodies, take with us all our collective life experiences and memories, and network them back into the life essence spirit energy network grid that is God, our creator. In this way, we serve our creator. Mother Nature and Father Sky have been talking to us for thousands of years to alter our path and reconnect with all animals. When Mother Nature is happy, she is creating enough oxygen to sustain life on this planet, and when Father Sky is happy, he gives us water and filters the sun for life to flourish. Thousands of years ago, our indigenous races knew this.

To begin our journey, we need to restore ourselves to our peak performance, so that we can resonate our correct frequency into Mother Earth and restore our place in the galaxy and in the cosmos. We need to start with improving our mind-body communication skills with our life vehicles, our transporters, and reconnect ourselves with our true spirit powers, our sixth senses. We do not pay our life vehicles enough attention, and we have not been responsible for our own self-care and well-being. We have the power and ability to slow our aging system down. Our sixth senses are an untapped resource that we are not aware of or taught about, and it allows life's energy to provide for us. We need to work with our spirit energy, not ignore or work against it. All evil comes from our disconnection from the spirit energy.

Our creator provided for us to be a part of the life essence spirit energy and God's protection. We have all been conditioned by our collective world consciousness from ancestor to ancestor with too many bad habits, routines, and beliefs that do not serve us and have become damaging to our well-being. One of the most important ones that has influenced and altered our physiology was encouraging us to becoming right-side conscious, so the majority of people on the planet use their right hand and leg as their dominant side, throwing our mental, physical, and spiritual programming out of balance. When we were designed, we were ambidextrous, using both sides of our bodies equally and easily. Now this leaves our left side to take on a support role, throwing off our programming. There are many things working against us at the moment, so it's time we become aware of them.

We need to start with ourselves first. We need to change our own values and attitudes, and we should show respect and empathy for ourselves and others. Changes internally can be made faster and can better serve us all, both now and for our future generations. This is our destiny. Our sixth senses are the greatest asset we have; without them, we would not have the power of free will, or the power of intention and attraction, to allow us to be creators in our own lifetime. Our creator bestowed upon us these great powers that are of the same image as God, and within the sixth sense's mcmory, they connect us to God directly with every design that our creator has fashioned in the book of creations, and that holds every answer and secret we have been looking for. Every invention or philosophy that we have created comes from a memory database, the life essence spirit memory set up by our creator. It's at our disposal, for us to become aware of, to focus on, and give it attention for it to appear in the physical.

When we are in tune with our sixth senses, all our dreams and expectations appear to those who are looking for them. We use the word *luck* very freely, however luck is not by accident. When opportunity and preparation meet, you have luck. Opportunities are around us every moment of every day, however we are not aware of them because we are not ready or prepared to see them. Whereas our repetitive negative emotions and thinking bring us stress and bad luck, a repetitive positive and optimistic outlook brings us opportunities, luck, happiness, and well-being. With hindsight, we can see through history the battle of good and bad forces. The more collective focus on good or bad gives us the outcome. Within our connection with our inner spirit, God, there is always good. In our self-conscious ego, there are many inner demons. Which one will you let win? your outcome relies on the one you feed the most. In order to fit into society, we sometimes allow our guards down, allowing ourselves to be manipulated and deceived, and to lower our values, morals, respect, and confidence. Only you can choose to be happy, good, righteous, and humane.

We have a responsibility to ourselves and to all life. The essence of life will restore our position in the balance of the universe. Earthlings are the caretakers of life, and through our collective consciousness, Mother Nature and Father Sky are talking to us. But are we listening? today the power of one energy involves manmade explosions, chemicals, and toxic waste in our rivers, oceans, and land. We're cutting down forests and jungles. These events have had a major effect on Mother Nature and the purity of our oxygen and ozone layer, or aura. This has created a chain reaction that has given us a lot of earthquakes, volcanic eruptions, and sinkholes all over the planet, shifting our seven major plates and our eight minor plates. It is more than global warming or climate change. Mother Nature is talking, and we are not listing or learning.

As usual, the minority and power mongers control our destiny and are destroying our planet. We will all suffer the consequences unless we stand up for our planet. Too often wc place our lives and well-being in the hands of others, who only give us temporary relief and benefits so that we are dependent on them. This devalues us and puts limitations on us and our confidence. Each one of us makes a difference. Collectively, we are the world consciousness.

Be cautious with what you think about and say. Control your emotions and have more empathy for life and the future of the human race. Walk the talk, stand proud, be happy, and assist others to be happy. Energy flows where attention goes.

May the essence be within you.

CHAPTER 7

FORCES THAT AFFECT YOUR LIFE VEHICLES

There are many beliefs on outside forces that affect our thoughts and emotions. By living in cities, we are disconnected from Mother Nature. Every day we walk on artificial surfaces and wear shoes that do not allow the earth to touch our skin. We have been conditioned to not get too dirty or play in Mother Nature, to be more hygienic, and to fear insects, spiders, cockroaches, and snakes. We find it difficult to go into Mother Nature because it requires an effort. We have become lazy, and only on weekends or holidays do we make an effort to enjoy Mother Nature and its healing effect on us.

I am not suggesting we walk around barefoot or roll around in the dirt, but we do need to make an effort to get among Mother Nature in order to connect and build our immune systems. Are you aware that we are bombarded every moment of every day with God's natural energy forces and manmade energy forces? All are running at different frequencies, and all energy forces are creating some type of energy field, EMF, or aura around the power source. These forces affect and dissect each other constantly, so how much do they affect you? No one is really sure, but let's look at both.

God's natural energy forces were fashioned and designed to assist us when they run at the correct harmonic default frequency setting that God set them at. However, if that setting is interfered with, the effects could be catastrophic. We know the sun and the moon affect our ocean tides every day, as we see on our news reports. Water is the body's principal chemical component, which makes up about 60 percent of the body's weight. Studies on full moons and their lunar effects have shown that it can alter individual behavior. Police and hospital workers have said it leads to more crime, trauma, and trouble sleeping.

We know all of God's creative designs were fashioned to serve and assist our very existence and evolution. Because we are the creator's sons and daughters, connected in his image, the Holy Spirit energy, we have to believe all these natural energy sources that God has fashioned would not cause us harm, if we respected them and used them wisely with faith. As we know, overexposure or overindulgence of anything is not good for us.

Electromagnetic fields are also formed by natural phenomena and geopathic stress lines, which are created by underground streams and cavities, mineral concentrations, and fault lines that are aggravated by manmade events, as well as alterations of the existing landscape with projects and constructions like cities, power stations, and explosions. As mere mortals, man is not sure or confident about any real outcome because we overuse, overestimate, and overindulge in everything we do. Greed and jealousy lead the way toward man's power race, not wisdom.

All manmade energy forces emit electromagnetic fields (EMFs) and are measured in Hertz, 1 cycle per second, like electricity that forms eddy currents. In Australia, electricity runs at 50 HZ, and there are also many other magnetic fields, like sound waves and radio and TV frequencies, which are all emitting frequencies around us twenty-four seven. Collectively they affect us and Mother Nature's natural harmonic frequencies. I do not expect any great changes to these sources and how we use them, however I would like you to be more aware of their effect on you. Regularly step out of them and make a conscious effort to cleanse yourself in Mother Nature's parks and beaches every day.

Every building we enter encases us with eddy currents and magnetic fields due to electrical cables in walls, ceilings, and floors. Then there are overhead and underground cables outside, running along every street to power all the buildings. Then there is all the TV, radio, mobile, and digital signals that run through the air, forming network grids that dissect each other. All of them collectively assist in raising our stress levels, causing headaches, fatigue, anxiety, insomnia, and muscle pain. We love our technology and luxuries, and it would be difficult to go without them, so let's become vigilant and protect ourselves and our loved ones. Let's take some responsibility for our well-being. When your mobile phones are on, use a hands-free set because they emit potential, harmful EMFs. Computer and laptops also emit EMFs, and the closer you are, the stronger the electromagnetic field. Travelling in cars, motorcycles, trains, and planes create their own EMFs. The electronics inside all appliances generate powerful, toxic EMFs. These fields can layer one upon the other, creating a harmful level of radiation. It's up to you to cleanse yourself mentally, physically, and spiritually.

I began my career as an electrician, data installer, and later service manager. I ran into various electromagnetic issues that we were not aware of then. I remember one incident in a high-rise building in the city, where a customer rang me with a problem that many other data experts could not solve. They had taken over a tenancy, fitting it out with an expensive data cabling network and equipment. However, when they carried out their initial tests, there were glitches on the computer screens and various other issues. On arrival, we carried out all the standard checks others had performed. I instructed my men to remove tiles in the ceiling to see whether there was any electrical interference from eddy currents above the system or running in parallel with the cables that could affect the network; it was all clear. Others had come and gone, and I knew I had to come up with something if I was to impress them and get further work.

I went to the floors below and above to investigate further. We found the issue: it was a large electrical switch board directly above the main data hardware. The electrical board above could not be moved, and the hardware physically could not be moved either, so what to do? I remembered in one of my data courses, it mentioned how EMFs would interfere with data signals. I told them I would come up with a solution but to give me a couple of day.

After pondering for a while, I realized I had to interfere with this EMF and break it. I decided to pick up some chicken mesh wire, screw it to the concrete ceiling directly under the electrical board, and connect a large electrical earth wire from the chicken mesh to the client's electrical switch board earth, to ground it. My boss thought I was crazy, and the client was angry and laughing at the same time. I had staked my reputation on a theory, however it worked, and they thought I was a genius. I received a lot of recommendations from this client; thank God it all paid off.

This was on only one floor of one building in the city, when the data world had just started going crazy. Massive hardware that took large areas of a building were used, and now there are smaller hardware and wireless signals. The amount of EMF interference is still felt every day by bad reception on our mobiles, TVs, radios, and internet signals. How much do they affect brainwave signals? Our brain wave signals change according to what we are doing and feeling. When our minds send out slower brain waves, we feel tired, lethargic, and dreamy. The higher frequency brain waves make us feel hyper alert. Brain wave speed is measured in Hertz, at one cycle per second. A normal human brain's frequency is 72 megahertz, and the human body is between 62–78 megahertz. Researchers at Taino Technology found that the human body becomes susceptible to colds and flu near 60 megahertz. The theory is if you can keep your body's frequency rate above 60 megahertz, you should rarely get sick.

There are six types of brainwaves: infra low, delta, theta, alpha, beta, and gamma. Infra low run below 0.5 Hz, and their slow nature makes them difficult to detect. They appear to take a major role in brain timing and network function. Delta brainwaves run at 0.5 to 3.0 Hz; they are slow, loud brainwaves, with a low frequency and deep penetrating, like a drumbeat. Theta brainwaves run at 3–8 Hz, and they occur most often in sleep and are dominant in deep meditation, learning, and memory. Here, our senses are withdrawn from the external world and are focused on signals originating from within our dream state, where we reach our sixth senses, intuition, and information beyond our normal conscious awareness. Where we also store our fears, troubled ancestral history, and nightmares.

Alpha brainwaves run at 8–12 Hz. It's the power of now, being present and aware. They also aid overall mental coordination, calmness, mind-body integration, and learning. Beta brainwaves run at 12–38 Hz and dominate our normal, awakened state of consciousness, our cognitive tasks, and the outside world. Beta is our fast activity when we are alert and attentive, solving problems, making decisions, and focused on mental activities. Running on high frequency is not an efficient way to run your brain because it takes up a lot of your energy. Gamma brainwaves run at 38–42 Hz and are the fastest of brainwaves. They work with simultaneous processing of information from different brain areas. They are highly active when in states of love, with an expanded consciousness, spirituality.

When our brainwaves are out of balance, there will be problems with our emotional or neurophysical health. An over arousal interference in certain brain areas can affect anxiety, anger, and aggression, whereas an under arousal in certain brain areas can lead to depression, attention deficit, chronic pain, and insomnia. It's believed a combination of both over arousal and under arousal is seen in cases of ADHD. Our self-conscious side of our brains determines our emotions, perceptions, and reactions to the world around us, strengthening or weakening our ability to repair our bodies and resist diseases. Our brains are capable of miraculous changes by eliminating uncomfortable patterns and restoring our systems to balance, allowing us to reach our peak performance, happiness, and well-being.

As for our manmade energy forces, with hindsight of our history, our collective world leaders have let us down. They choose to play games with our very existence. We are still prepared to think our way around everything without using or nurturing our natural instincts, our gut feeling, our natural sixth senses. These are able to provide us with the answers we need and require finding our true path back to our creator and immortality. We need to consciously remember that we are a Holy Spirit energy in a physical body and are in a virtual reality existence.

It's time we become aware of the true power of us and our unlimited capabilities when we are closer to God. We need to increase our natural aura around us so we can protect ourselves from all these electromagnetic fields interfering with our natural frequencies.

May the essence be within you.

CHAPTER 8

DNA AND PIXELS

Life is a reflection of itself. Every design our creator has fashioned in the book of creations shows the entire cosmos is made up of the life essence spirit memory. That memory is based on the circle, cells, dots, or default memory to allow everything to exist and hold its unique design in the big picture. For anything to function and hold its place, it needs a power source to sustain it. DNA are life memory cells, and their power source comes from our creator. It's the essence of life spirit energy that can never die. Similarly, pixels are digital memory cells, and their power source comes from manmade electricity. If the resources are there, they will never stop. Each can assist us in our evolution because they are the same sort of energy, a magnetic source but different.

All cells are represented by a circle. The circle of life is never ending and forever evolving. Any point on the circle could be where it starts, however there is no ending; it reignites and continues to evolve. DNA is a self-replicating material that is present in all living organisms, made up of cells with genetic information of fundamental and distinctive characteristics or qualities of someone or something. In a human, we usually refer to DNA as a drop of our blood, which replicates us physically, mentally, and emotionally with our routines, habits, and beliefs. Our flesh-and-blood body machine has every dot of its body sending and receiving information from our brains processing system instantaneously and twenty-four seven, for every thought and emotion, we have to generate an action and reaction from our bodies.

A pixel is generally thought of as the smallest single component of a digital image: a dot, a byte, a cell. In software, we are exposed to digital images all the time – computers, mobile phones, cameras, television, movies, virtual reality, and games. The number of pixels in an image is called the resolution, and the more pixels, the clearer the image.

Both pixels and DNA need a memory to evolve into a complete, creative image, and that image needs to be known or captured first for every dot to know their place in the big picture. Hence every dot needs the memory of the whole picture to hold its place.

In 1886, the French painter Georges Seurat used a technique called pointillism, which uses small, distinct dots of colour applied in patterns to form an image. Close up, the dots are clear, but when you stand back, the dots are not clear; it appears as a complete image.

In a digital image, collectively pixels create the complete image to appear as one. Computers run similar to our own minds: both have processors, memory banks, hard drives, files, default software settings, power sources, and allowances for updates to improve, protect, improvise, and restore defaults. However, every computer on this planet is no match to our minds' capabilities and processing systems. You are not aware of how much processing is required every minute of every day for your body machine, your life vehicle, to complete your daily routines and habits based on your ancestral and self-conscious beliefs, without any creativity added.

You are an intricate, unique being. Through our ancestral collective world consciousness, we have become stagnant, allowing ourselves to be caught in the deception of the rat race we call life. We are misled and misguided, allowing our inner demons, our emotions and constant self-talk, to create stress, anxiety, depression, fears, phobias, and addictions that control us. We need to activate our individual creativity and become aware of our inner power source and the life our creator gave us to live: as creators in his image with the essence of life, with the power of free will. Today, with technology we have ample knowledge available to us to start a better life, and it has assisted us in many ways thanks to our software designers' creativity, making everything in our lives easier to perform and achieve, so that we can communicate around the world with our mobiles and computers.

However, it has made us a lazier race, with a lack of communication and empathy toward others. There is a big difference between a human being and being human to sustain humanity. In the future, we need to go back to the basics and treat and respect others the way we want others to treat and respect us. Being human makes you an earthling who is a part of this living planet and everything in it. All is networked to God's life essence energy, the true power source. Everything on this planet has a power source and radiates its own energy field (aura) and frequency, to be defined in God's network. Collectively, everything on this planet creates one energy field to sustain life on our planet, including the ozone layer and earth's aura. Everything that has been designed and fashioned in the book of creations has its own energy field, aura, and frequency, to be defined individually in God's network, so every individual design knows the existence of every other design in the cosmos.

Each individual needs to step out of his ego self and reactivate his own life vehicle's frequency. Doing so will get you close up and personal with the true power of you, and it will network you back onto God's life grid. Everything we know or do is associated with pixels or cellular memory life cells; they are a reflection of each other, and a similarity makes them the same but different. We are still children in the universe. We should not be so hard on ourselves; there is still a lot to learn before we are ready to connect with the rest of the cosmos. The cosmos has always been aware of us, but we are not enlightened enough to see them even though they have always been among us.

May the essence be within you.

CHAPTER 9

YOU AND YOUR PERSONAL LIFE EXPERIENCES

Over my lifetime, I have met many great mentors and completed many courses on various topics: management, massaging, success coaching, life design, first aid, personal development, spiritual awareness, human behaviour, and electrical and data trade. I have also played a variety of sports, mainly rugby league, union, soccer, touch football, and surfing. I have had a pretty active lifestyle, like most people it is expected that after playing body contact sports and working in a trade a number of injuries can occur, every day people need operations, and others need rehabilitation with physiotherapy, chiropractic, and masseurs. There are also different types of illnesses, allergies, and diseases you can pick up or pass on. From your ancestors' DNA; you can get them from birth, and they stay with you till the day you die.

All these issues have a dramatic effect on your mental and physical traumas and stresses, creating anxiety, depression, and addiction to prescription drugs for pain. You seek social drugs and alcohol to escape from your immediate issues, using coffee or cigarettes to calm your nerves. As we have become aware in previous chapters, whatever goes in your mind affects your thoughts and emotions, clouding your judgment and actions, which directly affect your mind-body communication and causes tension and strain to your muscle memory and body functions. As human beings, we are constantly bombarded in every environment. Our bodies have their own pharmacy, constantly creating chemicals to support our white blood cells to combat against our bodies' enemies. We have hormones and endorphins that decrease pain, burn fat, build muscle, increase bone density, and sharpen our alertness.

We have all heard about the placebo effect and how it is used to trick the ego, the self-conscious, to think what we are given will cure our issues or illnesses. This is a simple method to clear your mind of any doubts and fears to allow your body to heal itself. First you need to believe the source who is giving you the remedy is one you can trust. This is a prime example of the power of free will, which you have at your disposal and do not know how to use correctly. The power of free will is a part of every thought you have, and all your outcomes are determined by your intentions and the emotions you place around them. The human body machine's DNA recipe is running an automatic program before you are even born, and it already has the cellular memory of everything about you physically, mentally, and spiritually: your ancestral files, your creator's default files, and a set of files that are ready to gather information as your self-consciousness or ego files when you are activated in your mother's womb. You're continuously gathering information with your five natural senses and your spiritual sixth senses throughout your life.

As a child there are many falls, illnesses, and traumas that are deemed unimportant at the time. However, as you grow, all these experiences can and will affect your postural alignment as you grow into an adult. When you hit your twenties and your skeletal frame is at its strongest, your body's muscle memory is connected like vines around your skeletal frame. They are part of set muscle groups that make you a Homo sapiens, however each group is segregated by your seven major skeletal joints, where your muscle memory can twist any joint, affecting your alignment and well-being.

Learning to become aware of your twisted muscles and joints allows you to practice Destressercise. Using your normal, sedentary movements you can do some body shaping and become your own mind-body mentor and self-healer. Unusual events and things can happen in our lives. In my early twenties, I developed my first and only allergy, a seafood allergy that has on several occasions created near-death experiences, each stronger than the previous. Through all of these experiences, I have had a number of epiphanies and insights, which I have shared with you in this book. I finally narrowed it down from seafood to prawns. It almost killed me, but I can still eat crabs, lobsters, mussels, and oysters. During my last episode, I thought I had died. Surprisingly, I was very calm and relaxed, when I awoke my face looked like I had gone ten rounds with Muhammad Ali, and the swelling took a week to go down. I avoid prawns altogether now. The funny thing is before my first prawn allergy, I had eaten prawns many times without a reaction. Our bodies can react to anything at anytime.

My outlook, awareness, and perceptions were different after those near-death experiences, and I felt like I was detached from others and did not fit in. I was playing rugby at that time with the boys' mentality around me and plenty of support and friends, but I found myself alone and isolated from them, my family, and my other friends. Through a female friend, I found myself going to spiritual awareness classes, where normally only woman went. I pursued more knowledge about my intuition and psychic powers, but I was too scared to talk about it, so I tried to blend in, playing my sports and trying to be normal.

Everyone can look back at a number of setbacks, injuries, illnesses, and misfortunes that affected them mentally and physically. In hindsight, they can make us stronger or weaker depending on what belief system we have to support us. I was taught to pay more attention, listen to my gut feelings and instincts, create an optimistic positive belief system that will never let me down, be my own best friend, and love myself without limitations. Always remember that "energy flows where attention goes." Be cautious on what you regularly focus your attention. The last two years have pushed my limits. I tore a old muscle injury in my right rotator cuff, making it three times bigger than it was. I was originally advised I didn't need to stitch it up and that physiotherapy and resistive training would strengthen it. For a few years, it seemed okay, however it tore again.

While I was waiting for my insurance to approve worker's compensation and an operation, I was on light duties. I had another unfortunate accident, where a wall on a burnt-out site collapsed, while my hand was resting on top of a step ladder, a slab of bricks landed on my left hand's first finger after my thumb and crushed the bone to dust. The slab miraculously bounced over my shoulder and missed the rest of my body. I was lucky to be alive. I was told the finger could not be saved, so it was amputated. After a seven-month period, I went in for my shoulder operation. I was recovering from injuries on my left and right side.

Unfortunately, it didn't stop there. After some of the swelling on my left hand went down, I had difficulty moving my other fingers and had to have another operation on the elbow, to reposition a nerve that had moved from shock and was stretched to the max. I had three operations in less than two years. I had painful feelings all over, scar tissue, and trauma in my muscle memory, locking up my fingers, wrists, elbows, shoulders, neck, back, hips, and legs. I was not in good shape.

I went to physiotherapy twice a week, as recommended. It was only twenty minutes a session, so forty minutes a week was supposed to heal me? There was no relief, so I decided I would get some massages as well. They assisted me, but I needed to do more. The pain and tension was always there, and the more aware I became of the pain and my muscle memory, the more I could relieve it. Fortunately, I had unknowingly prepared myself with my mind-body communication skills, my massage experience, my spiritual awareness techniques, my optimistic attitude, and the phrase "Energy flows where attention goes." I worked diligently on my injuries, creating routines and habits around all my joints to relieve and release some pain. I combined a lot of these techniques and realized that meditation did not have to be in complete silence, and I did not have to clear my mind of thoughts. I simply had to move my thoughts and focus on where I needed it. I would constantly focus my attention and work on my seven joints as often as possible. It got to a point that people would notice what I was doing and ask me why I was doing it all the time. I established a mind-body communication that released trapped trauma and scar tissue to allow deep cellular muscle tissue to start healing. I used closing my eyes, focusing on my joints with controlled breathing, and massaging that area. That made a dramatic effect, and then I tried the same method without closing my eyes and found it still worked. As a masseur, I have found the majority of people ignore their pain and only get minimal treatment; they don't want to deal with pain and prefer to take something to temporarily relieve it. It's all mind over matter. The majority of people deal with pain no matter how minor, even a headache every day; they get used to it and accept it, so it never leaves them alone. Addictions are connected to pain as well; whether mental, emotional, or physical, most people believe any relief is good, and they consume themselves in the addiction.

I would like to share with you my Destressercise mind-body awareness self-healing program in order to help you have a more fulfilled and healthier life. All you need to know is that in your subconscious files, I can direct you though the right mind-body pathways to self-awareness and mindfulness, in order to release and control your pain. You can successfully overcome stress and find the true power of you and the life you were meant to live, which is your destiny. You and I are a reflection of our inner source. The true power of you is a divine power that we all share with our creator. It's a self-healing power that our life vehicles are programmed to perform. The only restriction is you – your ego's negative self-talk and emotions. My legacy is to assist you with Destressercise in order to get you close up and personal with your muscle memory and the true power of you, your sixth senses.

The unity and healing of the human race is in our hands; it's our birthright, it is in our DNA makeup, and it is an energy that sustains the essence of life and the source to our divine power. It's a power of one that is the power of you and the power of all living beings, networked together to evolve into our true destinies in the life essence spirit virtual reality.

CHAPTER 10

DESTRESSERCISE: A MIND-BODY SELF-HEALING AWARENESS PROGRAM

Destressercise takes you on the ultimate virtual reality mind-body-spirit experience. It uses self-hypnosis meditation techniques to get you close up and personal with the true power of you. You can establish new empowering mind habits, new awareness body habits, and new enlightening spirit habits to support and guide yourself.

In our new world of technology, we always say we are time poor, but we have plenty of time to get on the phone, the iPad, or the computer to chat, surf the web, or play a game. Why not access your own ultimate virtual reality game, which allows you to place your self-consciousness into a self-hypnosis meditation? Use your third eye to guide you through a mind, body, and spirit journey that you will never forget! Destressercise techniques take you on a journey to unleash the true power of you and reveal your sixth senses, which connect you to your natural instincts, paternal and maternal instincts, gut feeling, intuition, psychic ability, self-healing powers, telekinesis, levitation, and Holy Spirit energy. It's your life essence virtual reality software.

By focusing on changing the images, thoughts, and emotions in your mind, you give yourself a new outcome. By focusing entirely on your inner Holy Spirit and mind-body communication, with the philosophy that energy flows where attention goes, you become more creative and stimulated. Destressercise takes you on a guided close up and personal connection with your cellular and muscle memory. Be kind to your auto conscious memory and release the pain and stress attached to every cell and dot (pixel) of your body. Your mind, your processor, has a direct connection to every cell, and needle dot of your body instantaneously, so take advantage of it. Destressercise takes your everyday, sedentary habits and gets you to create repetitious movement and focus around your essential body mechanics seven major joints. Doing this on an everyday basis can release tension and pain, creating new routines and beliefs that serve you and improve your well-being. It is normal for you to want to know where your life path is taking you. You simply need to listen to your life essence spirit memory, the Holy Spirit, that has all the wisdom and information you need for a successful, healthy, and enlightened life. All of this has been available to you from the beginning of time; it lies within your subconscious and your spirit's default files. These files are a manual for you to improve yourself, honour your true values, and follow your destiny.

Destressercise uses your essential body mechanics as a stress-relieving, self-healing awareness program to help you take control and responsibility of your well-being and self-care. Too often we place our well-being in the hands of others, who give us temporary relief and dependency on them. That devalues you and puts limitations on yourself, decreasing self-confidence and belief. Based on a set of balanced, conscious movements designed to release the tension in muscles throughout the body, Destressercise uses circular movements based on the circle of life, where movements are performed by rotating clockwise and anticlockwise at the seven major joints of the body; these joints are where tension is stored.

It starts at the feet, the base of your life vehicle's body tower and symmetry, to stimulate blood flow and self-healing. Just like a body builder builds muscles by focusing on individual muscle groups (which tears muscle tissue, stimulating fresh blood to the area to increase muscle mass), there is only one body-building exercise that uses the term *concentration,* and that's the concentration curls. They're used to increase the biceps muscle mass by restricting movement to only the bicep using a controlled weight, visual awareness, and focus to stimulate blood to the area and enhance that muscle. By connecting to your mind-body communication, Destressercise uses your essential body mechanics to incorporate these methods and various other techniques to its program. No weights or strenuous activities are required, however as you advance, you can adapt them to any exercise, sport, job, or event.

Some of the other awareness techniques used are the left-brain, right-brain techniques, adopting more ambidextrous habits that are used to reactivate dormant muscle tissues our brains' belief systems have prerecorded through our routine sedentary movements, habits, and experiences. Our subconscious programming has altered and shifted our posture to suit a dominant side of our body, from right to left and from bottom to top. This does not serve us, so the three steps we must take uses our brains' instantaneous mind-body communication, networking us to every dot in our body to our conscious advantage. The first step is improving your awareness of your postural alignment and how your mental self-chatter affects your wellbeing. Second, you place focus on the muscles surrounding your seven essential body mechanics and the major joints individually. Third, you create a repetitious attention with intention to heal them.

Before being born, our bodies, minds, spirits, and ancestral DNA memories have recorded and registered trauma, shock, and stress. As an infant and through our childhood, our skeletal frames are fragile and growing and don't reach full growth and strength till we reach our teens. We are more dependent on our muscular structure to support our bodies' frames, through the most active, emotional, and sensitive times of our lives, until our skeletal frames catch up. Our minds, through our intricate and precise nervous systems, are controlling all our muscles, emotions, experiences, and positive or negative self-talk, recording and storing information into our subconscious minds. Did you know that 70 percent of our lives is spent in the subconscious automind, with thoughts that make up all our habits, routines, beliefs, and attitudes like an autopilot? They are manifested into our bodies' muscle tissues by our subconscious minds. it has no malice and doesn't know any better; it simply runs a programming system. We are only restricted and sick as the prerecorded inner secrets in our subconscious minds files. Only we are responsible for the knowledge and information we receive, analyze, and record in our subconscious auto programming, which makes us who we are today. We are as healthy as the communication between our mind, body, and spirit.

How good is your communication? No one is to blame for where you are and what has been stored in your subconscious autopilot. All people are dealing with issues and events with the knowledge they have attained over their lifetimes, as well as past generations of knowledge stored in cellular memory.

The power of using Destressercise and your essential body mechanics takes you back to the basics, teaching you how to use a blueprint of intention, to one point of focused concentration that gives gratitude and appreciation for the *power of you.* Forgive yourself, release all fears and limitations, and open your inner self and conscious mind to receive the gift that has been waiting to be opened since you were born.

The secret that will give you total happiness, well-being, youthfulness, passion, and success in your life has been right under your nose. It's based on the 30 percent factor, It is only in the 30 percent conscious filtered time that we can stop what is going into our subconscious. It's the window of opportunity to go in and change any of the old, stored body stress recordings, which we now feel do not fit with our real image and purpose. All these manifestations from the day we were born twist and distort the muscle fibers, which cling to the skeletal frame and pull it from its naturally balanced alignment.

Imagine as an infant, your body muscle structure has an auto protection system, an autoimmune system, an auto healing system, and your own pharmacy that is dependent on your well-being, without a supportive skeletal frame that only reaches its full strength in your teens. How well aligned do you think that muscular structure will allow the skeletal structure to fit in? It is only at your seven major (and various minor) joints that adjustments can be made to form good or bad posture. In your body's gradual growth, you and your subconscious mind think you are in balance and working perfectly, with no problems. It's only in your mature conscious you become aware of challenges, traumas, and injuries that bring you out of alignment through pain, anger, fears, and limitations.

We cannot be totally dependent on others and outside sources to resolve all our issues. A stable environment is a must. However, if you do not personally allocate part of that 30 percent conscious time to all areas of your life (health, relationships, career, finances) and have a one-on-one with yourself to find the truth about the real you and release the true power of you, then you will remain stagnant in the 70 percent subconscious life you unknowingly inherited, created, and live.

We are God's children, given the abundant and divine power of creators. We were made in his image, and the creative God consciousness sustains all life on our planet and beyond. We are always searching in the wrong places for the answers to our creation and purpose. As the children of God, it lies within us, and only we can take that journey with ourselves to reach the creative spirit consciousness that lies within the soul of our physical bodies and connects us to the God consciousness that has all the knowledge and answers we seek. We have been created in this physical body and dimension to realign our minds, bodies, and spirits to be connected as one. The power of one is our test and challenge in faith. It is through the intimate mind-body experience that we open our physical antennas that connect us through the soul to our inner spirits. We are all intuitive beings; it's only our physicality and ego that gets in the way. We have to remember we are living spiritual beings in physical bodies, and we have roles to play. Rather than our egos and attitudes controlling our lives, we need to stand up and be accountable and responsible for our actions.

Every human body has created with its mind-body experiences a unique, twisted muscular mass structure that contains the skeletal frame in its present state. We have always had the ability to change that state. No matter how old we are, we are still children of God, and with the curiosity, innocence, and naivety of children, it will always remain within us. It is that same inner consciousness that will restore our youthfulness, well-being, passion, and zest for life and love, which is a natural instinct that we require to reach our higher purpose. The creative God consciousness is the same consciousness we all use at this present moment, and throughout the evolution of human life, we have always strived to raise our level of consciousness. We now stand at a moment of time that requires us to become aware of our responsibility as God's caretakers and green keepers of all life, and to begin the journey and raise our levels of consciousness as the power of one. We should use the correct intentions to restore our global consciousness, based on love and forgiveness to ourselves and all living beings, as well as attracting the universal abundance of knowledge and energy that the oneness makes available to us in order to sustain life for eternity.

I believe 2018 will realign an awakening, a window of consciousness, that will take us to places we have only dreamed of and created as stories. We are at a milestone of scientific and spiritual discoveries that will propel us into a creative, conscious future for the benefit of all life, and we need to be prepared. The opportunity is here right now. Luck is something we all wish we had more of. When opportunity and preparation meet, you have luck. How prepared are you? Are you willing to find the true you and restore your place in the universal God consciousness? Let's do it! It starts with you.

Destressercise has designed the use of your essential body mechanics to get you close up and personal with the true power of you. Using the window of the 30 percent factor, Destressercise provides you with a mind-body self-healing awareness programmed for your preventative maintenance to realign your body's symmetry and create balance and harmony in your state of physiology. No matter how minor your stress may be at the moment and how well you think you have controlled it, you have had years of unknowingly manifested stress in your body. A body being out of alignment will always instigate some type of chain reaction that affects the skeletal frames position, starting from the feet and moving up through the hips and pelvis, the centre of our support structure, and all the way up to the neck.

You may say we can change the postural skeletal frame through chiropractors, or manipulate the muscles through physiotherapy and massages. These are all good treatments. Destressercise compliments and supports these treatments. However, the muscle fibers that hold our frames out of balance throughout our lives is more than just physical. We manifested tension, trauma, and stress from our stored subconscious memories, sending it into our bodies. Only we can consciously change that program, and any assistance is a bonus.

Our mind has an automatic protection system to adjust or supply what is required to keep the body sustained. Even as far as shifting more weight from one side to the other to let the body function, this movement also affects the nervous system, blood flow, and all body organs, causing all types of dis-ease, ailments, and severe issues. Only the programmer, you, can consciously go to each physical joint and muscle group, on a regular routine, to deactivate these tensions and stresses deep in your body structure. This brings new meaning to being health conscious.

In order to bring balance to your physiology and place you in a positive state, Destressercise has designed a simple mat for your brain to become aware of your true parameters. You can record your present body symmetry so that you can consciously create the window of the 30 percent factor to correct and realign your base tower at your feet, which are the foundations of your body's tower. The mat is made up of horizontal and vertical lines, creating squares approximately five millimeters apart for better accuracy. Your mind uses true alignments as reference points.

Place your feet on the mat and then line up the tips of your big toes on one of the horizontal lines and the side of your big toes and heels on the vertical line, to straighten both feet. Start with your knees bent, back straight, and head looking forward and slightly up. Close your eyes and focus. Slowly straighten your knees and become aware of any imbalance, tension, or pain; let your mind check your new readings with your existing subconscious files. If you feel giddy or strange, open your eyes, hold the position, and try again to close your eyes until you feel comfortable. The more you create a repetitious routine around this, the more your mind will acknowledge your true alignments and alter your default alignment to the true one.

If you do not have a mat, you can use any tiled floor or lines. However, your mat can be taken anywhere with you, even into Mother Nature. Hydration is a must, so drink a glass of water before you start, and have water near you at all times. Destressercise uses controlled breathing techniques that allow you to maximize your inner experience. We start at our feet with the Destressercise mat so that our essential body mechanics are easy to see and define with the lines. Then we move on to our backs with some floor movements before finishing on our feet without the mat and defined lines to allow our conscious and subconscious minds to coordinate and realign. This needs to be repeated regularly for it to become a default new setting.

Start slowly, and be light and nimble, slowly increasing speed, stretching muscle tissues around the seven major joints with a circular motion both clockwise and anticlockwise. Start with your dominant side and then the other, to assess movement on both sides. Use the dominant side as a reference point to bring your other side to respond with the same movements. Then move both sides together in unison. Use this kind of basic stretch routine with low impact repetition and stretch movements for loosening, revitalizing, strengthening, and healing the body's muscles and joints.

Focus your mind on every move. A pinpoint concentration is required through your natural mind-body communication in order to feel your body's movements and sense your body's tension. The use of controlled, deep breathing (in through your nose and out through your mouth) helps realign your body's true postural symmetry. Energy flows where attention goes.

As a mind-body self-awareness and self-healing programme, Destressercise was designed for all human beings. No matter what body shape, fitness condition, or age you are, anyone can do it and benefit from the results. So let's do it! The transition from your normal self-consciousness or ego's body awareness to your new self-awareness and mind, body, and spirit communication brings balance and harmony back under your control. Destressercise techniques improve your awareness, attention, and focus to develop your mind-body communication skills by using your essential body mechanics and the seven major joints as reference points. Only you can successfully alter your existing muscle memory in order to improve your postural alignment and rhythmically balance and harmonise your body. Mind-body communication skills guide you to mentally pinpoint your weaknesses and pain, reawaken your brain signals to your muscle and joint memory, relax the mind, and relieve stress from your muscle memory so you can feel young and full of vitality.

As we consciously take the journey to map out our trapped tensions and focus on a particular point, we send a harmonic frequency from our brains through our nervous systems, which automatically send fresh blood to that area, breaking down tense fibers, scare tissue and increasing blood flow to make the muscle fibers suppler and encourage self-healing.

You need to first find your pain. Nurture it, befriend it, and love it in order to fix it. Your body will love you and heal itself. Don't ever ignore your pain or leave it alone, Your life vehicle is your responsibility, and it becomes your top concern over everything but God. Only you can release your potential and bring passion into your life.

Destressercise uses your mind-body communication and your natural instincts to get you close up and personal with the true power of you. It uses your essential body mechanics and the seven major joints as reference points. It is designed to assist you with your self-care and self-healing via a body mechanics maintenance plan.

The Destressercise philosophy is "Energy flows where attention goes." It strives to support you to successfully overcome stress and release your pain in order to begin a healthy mind, body, and spirit life.

May the Essence Be Within You

Printed in the United States
By Bookmasters